Paleo For Beginners

Intro and tips to get you started The Paleo way

AMARPREET SINGH

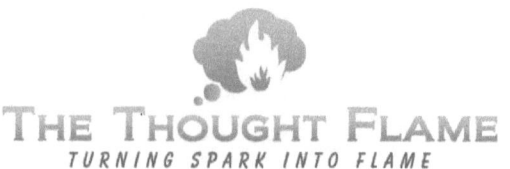

THE THOUGHT FLAME
TURNING SPARK INTO FLAME

info@thethoughtflame.com

www.thethoughtflame.com

Table of Contents

Introduction

Walking into a supermarket sometimes can be a little overwhelming. It can be difficult even for the best of us to pinpoint which foods are healthy among the sea of shiny and clean packages of food within a supermarket. It can be even more difficult when you are trying to keep yourself and your family as healthy as possible. Every day we are abused by an onslaught of ads via the TV, internet, radio and in magazines of the different junk foods and so called "healthy meals" out there that it can be hard to tell the difference between the truly healthy meals and the so called "new fad diets."

What has come from all of this pointless advertisement? An increasing number of people or are overweight including mean, women and children. So how can you tell what is really healthy for you when you are mind-blown by the number of choices out there? Simply go on the Paleo Diet.

If you are new to the Paleo Diet then this is exactly the book that you will need. In this guide you will learn a variety of things such as what foods you should avoid eating, how to stay healthy with the foods that you eat in the long run and how to simplify the entire process. Lastly you will find an array of healthy and delicious Paleo friendly recipes that will help easy you away from unhealthy foods so you can live the healthy and long life that you deserve.

So, let's not waste any more time. Let's get started already!

Chapter One: What Is The Paleo Diet?

Whether you are new to the Paleo diet or not, know that the Paleo diet is not just another fashion trend diet. It is in fact a lifestyle choice that can help transform you and your body into exactly what you want it to be: healthy and fit. This diet is solely based on the lifestyle and diet habit of our ancient ancestors who were around before the time of agriculture

Remember, during this time there were many people who lived solely to hunt and gather what food they could and if they couldn't find anything, they didn't eat. Whatever our ancestors could get their hands on is what they ate and what they ate they did so in its purest form such as vegetables, a variety of fresh fruit, eggs, plenty of meat, fish and seeds.

It is because this type of food that the human body was able to act so efficiently for so many years. However, in our current time with the advances in culture, medicine and technology the food that we consume has changed dramatically and while are bodies are able to adapt to these changes quite nicely, this harmful food has still managed to ravage our bodies in ways that we never knew possible before.

The Benefits of The Paleo Diet

While you have probably heard many people hype about this type of diet, it is still no secret how unhealthy processed foods are for your body. Many dieticians and nutritionists agree that the best diet for you is one that is as pure as possible as that is what our bodies are naturally used to. In this section you will learn of the most popular benefits of this diet and see why this diet is great for you.

1. Improve Your Overall Nutrition-with this diet you are consuming food is their most natural state and this state helps to provide you with a variety of nutrients and minerals that you would otherwise not get with processed foods.

2. Increase In Nutrient Absorption-when you remove all of the harmful ingredients from food such as artificial ingredients and harmful toxins, your body is able to absorb all of the nutrients it needs much better.

3. Lose Weight In The Process-with the Paleo diet, you use ingredients that incredibly healthy for you. Using whole foods in this diet that consist of a higher number of nutrients that you need will help you to burn much more fat in the process while helping you to take in less calories than you would with processed foods.

4. Help To Improve Digestion-this is the main reason that the Paleo diet is very popular. The Paleo Diet helps to remove irritating grains from your system as well as improve your overall gut health. It also helps to keep you regular in the long run.

Chapter Two: A Few Tips For New Paleo Dieters

Starting something new can be both exciting and very scary all at the same time. However, there are a few things that many Paleo dieters should all know and consider before fully committing to this lifestyle and in this chapter you will learn for yourself what helpful tips you will need in order to be a successful Paleo Dieter.

1. Have An Open Mind

There is no way faster to failure than having a certain way of negative thinking and attitude towards your new diet. This cannot be any truer for the Paleo diet and lifestyle and this is something that is not going to be easy for many people to commit to. Try to think very positive about this endeavor. If you go into it thinking that you are just punishing yourself and that it will not last forever, trust me it won't. That is the kind of thing that you want to avoid.

2. If Cooking At Home, Make Sure You Give Yourself Plenty of Time To Do So

There is nothing worse than making a fresh home cooked meal and having to rush through it. While it may seem like this is not going to be hard to do, arranging meals around vegetables will be a foreign concept for many people and it will take them several minutes to do and to get right the first time. Give yourself plenty of time to do this and you will be able to create hearty and delicious meals that will leave you feeling satisfied.

3. Avoid Any Type of Convenience Food

If you are skeptical about how delicious or savory Paleo dishes can be, I highly recommend that you stay away from as many convenience food products as possible. Trust me, I have yet to taste one type of convenience food that has been healthy and that I liked really well. If you think that you will be able to live on frozen pizza, frozen Paleo burritos and veggie burger patties every single day, you are going to be in one heck of a surprise.

4. Do Not Be Embarrassed About Living This Kind of Lifestyle

There may come a time where you will feel that you have to rationalize your decision or explain your decision to other people. You may even find yourself coming up with reasons behind your Paleo lifestyle such as, "I'm doing it as a research project or I don't want to be unhealthy anymore." Regardless of what reason you are using, you will begin to notice the same thing happening over and over again: explaining yourself never feels good.

Never feel that you have to explain your decision to anybody. However, if you do want something to tell people I find it easy to come out and say, "I have always agreed with Paleo philosophy and this just felt right." Most people have nothing to say to that statement. In fact most people will become more intrigued and you will find yourself having an interesting discussion with people that you may or may not know.

5. Don't Be Afraid of The Produce Isle

Going Paleo means that you will get to become close and personal with the produce isle then you may have been before. Once you start this diet is a good idea to head down this isle to learn and explore exactly what your new diet will begin to consist of. Look at how much diversity you have with plants and try to come up with some creative meal ideas while surrounded by the main ingredients that you will be using.

11

6. Stay As Strong As You Possibly Can

Going Paleo is not the easiest thing that you will ever do. In fact, it will be one of the hardest things that you will do. The first few days will be especially tough on you, but I promise it does become easier as days pass. You will soon get into the swing of things and living this lifestyle will become easier and easier. It will come to a point that when you think of what you want to make for every meal, meat will never cross your mind.

7. When In Doubt, Stick With Simplicity

Just because you are a Paleo dieter and you are using vegetable and healthy meats to make up the majority of your meals, it does not mean that you have to make the entire process complicated. The best recipes to make are the simple ones and not only will you enjoy these recipes, but so will your guests.

If you are just starting out on the Paleo Diet, these helpful tips will help you to become a successful Paleo dieter in the long run. Whether you ensure to explore your options when eating out, staying as strong as possible with your new lifestyle, having an open mind about being a Paleo Dieter, making sure that you stay clear of convenience foods and making sure to give yourself plenty of time to prepare your meals, make sure that you try to follow these tips every once in a while. You will become a better Paleo dieter for it in the long run.

Chapter Three: How To Make Your Meals Taste Better

When it comes to eating a Paleo diet most of the time people are hesitant about it. Why is this? The main reason people are resistant to the idea of eating a healthy Paleo diet is because many people are under the misconception that the food will not taste as good as a regular fast food burger and fries will. This is one of the most popular misconceptions regarding a Paleo diet today and in my opinion it is one that stops many people from becoming great Paleo dieter and from living a healthier lifestyle in the long run.

When you first begin preparing Paleo food, many people do not know how to make their dishes tastes good. There are so many different flavors to work with that bringing them out so that you can savor them can be extremely difficult. There are many different seasoning that you can use to bring out the flavor of your dish and to help impress not only yourself, but your friends and family as well.

Here are a few different tips that you can use to help make your Paleo meals taste more amazing and to get you excited to prepare your meals on a daily basis.

1. Make Sure That You Use Only High-Quality and Fresh Ingredients

One of the best ways to ensure that your food tastes just as delicious as possible is to ensure that you are using the highest quality ingredients that you can afford and that you are as fresh as possible.

If you are the type of person who usually only spends enough money to get the cheapest ingredients possible, you will begin to notice that you meals are lacking in flavor, making it more possible that you will stop your Paleo diet before you want to.

I highly recommend using fresh organic ingredients, as they always tend to pack more punch then ordinary produce. Keep in mind, the ingredients that are simple and that are not stuffed with things like salt and sugar, have more flavor and will help your meals to taste delicious in the long run.

2. Don't Be Afraid To Spice Things Up

Using different herbs and spices should start becoming a regular part of your meal preparing process and it is something that you should get in the habit of adding into your meals on a daily basis. Not only do herbs and spices help to add incredible flavor to your meals, but many of them are packed with important nutrients that your body needs on a daily basis.

Some of the most popular and great tasting spices that you can use are turmeric, cinnamon, cumin and ginger. These four spices can help liven up a dull Paleo dish and can even help benefit your body in the long run such as by giving your digestive system a boost that it desperately needs.

Using fresh herbs in your dishes can also help give your body important antioxidants and nutrients that it needs. Herbs like Parsley, cilantro, Basil and Mint can be used for much more then great tasting garnishes and you can use them for a variety of reasons in your main dishes.

3. When Using Beans and Grains, Give Them A Boost Once In A While

If you have ever eaten plain chickpeas or brown rice, you know better than anybody how unappealing they can be. They are completely bland and don't really have much of a taste to them. If you are making a dish that must incorporate these two ingredients, I highly recommend that you do not serve them on their own.

I highly recommend pairing your beans and grains with ingredients that are rich in flavor. Try mixing them with some of your favorite pieces of fruit. There are even some vegetables that you can use that can help liven up the flavors of these otherwise bland foods.

I also recommend adding a healthy helping of flavorful sauce or dressing to some of these ingredients.

4. Don't Be Afraid To Use Fat In Your Meals

While choosing the right kind of fat to use in your dish is important to keep your meals and yourself as healthy as possible, the more you do it, the easier the process becomes down the line. Adding healthy forms of fat not only have healthy benefits for you, but it can go a long way into making your meals much more delicious. Fat carries the richness of the entire dish and can make or break how the dish will taste to you and your family.

There are many types of healthy fat that you can use to enhance the flavor of your dish such as fats coming from whole foods like seeds, avocados, olives and nuts. If you find that you are preparing a meal for other people who are following the Paleo lifestyle as well, it will help to add a healthy form of fat to enhance the taste of dish.

5. Don't Be Afraid To Use Salt Here and There

Salt helps out to bring out the flavor of important Paleo friendly ingredients such as vegetables and even helps to soften them a bit whenever you are cooking them up or sautéing them. When you are preparing your meals do not be afraid to add as much salt as you want to help bring out the flavor of your veggies.

If you are afraid of taking in too much sodium there are healthy alternatives that you can use to help enhance the flavor of your dishes. Don't be afraid to use vegetable salt every once in a while as it contains lots of important nutrients and less sodium than regular table salt.

I know that starting a Paleo diet can be very scary and can even feel intimidating when you do not believe that you will be able to eat delicious meals again. However, there are certain things that you can do to enhance the flavors of your dishes such as using salt, healthy forms of fat or using fruits to bring out the flavors of your dishes. Follow these helpful tips to make the most delicious Paleo friendly recipes you will ever make in your life.

Chapter Four: Delicious Paleo Diet Recipes

What is a Paleo Cookbook without some healthy and nutritious Paleo diet recipes? In this chapter you will discover a variety of healthy Paleo diet recipes that you can put together for breakfast, lunch or dinner and enjoy a new lifestyle that you deserve.

Vegetable and Ham Early Morning Frittata

It is no secret that breakfast is one of the most important meals of the day. With this recipe you can ensure that you get your early morning feast that not only tastes great, but looks great as well.

Makes: 4 Servings

Ingredients:

-8 Eggs, Large In Size and Beaten Lightly

-2 Cups of Spinach, Fresh and Finely Chopped

-1 Tomato, Medium In Size and Finely Chopped

-1/2 Onion, Yellow and Thinly Sliced

-1/2 Red Bell Pepper, Thinly Sliced

-1 Tbsp. of Coconut Oil

-Dash of Salt and Pepper For Taste

Directions:

1. Using a large sized skillet, heat it up over medium to high heat. At the same time preheat your oven to a broil.

2. Add in your onions, peppers, salt and pepper to your skillet and allow to cook for 3 minutes until the vegetables become tender. Make sure that you stir constantly. Then add in your tomato and spinach and allow to cook for 2 minutes or until the spinach becomes wilted.

3. Next pour in your beaten eggs and begin to stir as gently as possible.

4. Then transfer your hot skillet into your oven and allow to cook until the eggs begin to set and the top begins to brown. Remove from the oven and allow to sit for 3 minutes until you serve.

Creamy Broccoli Soup

If you are looking for a soup recipe that will leave you feeling full and satisfied, this is the perfect soup recipe for you. Creamy in texture and absolutely delicious, this dish will leave you craving more.

Makes: 4 Bowls

Ingredients:

-1 Tbsp. of Coconut Oil

-8 Cups of Broccoli, Florets Only

-1 Cup of Cauliflower, Florets Only

-1 Tbsp. of Garlic, Minced

-4 Cups of Chicken Broth, Organic

-1 Onion, Yellow, Medium In Size and Chopped Finely

-Dash of Salt and Pepper For Taste

-2 Tbsp. of Coconut Butter

-1 Cup of Coconut Milk, Unsweetened

Directions:

1. Using a medium sized soup pot, heat up a touch of oil over medium to high heat. Add in your broccoli first, then cauliflower and onion. Allow to cook for the next 6 to 8 minutes or until it begins to get tender.

2. Next stir in your garlic and allow to cook for one minute. Last add in your remaining ingredients and allow mixture to come to a boil.

3. Reduce your heat to low and allow the soup to simmer for 20 minutes or until the vegetables are fully tender.

4. Then remove from heat and puree the soup in a blender until smooth in consistency. Serve immediately and enjoy.

Dairy Free Salad

Who doesn't enjoy a salad ever now and then? With this recipe you can enjoy a tasty and light salad that will leave you feeling refreshed and healthy at the same time.

Makes: 4 Servings

Ingredients:

-3/4 Cup of Coconut Milk, Canned

-1/4 Cup of Tahini, Sesame

-Dash of Salt and Pepper For Taste

-2 Tbsp. of Lemon Juice, Fresh

-10 Cups of Romaine Lettuce, Fresh and Chopped Roughly

-1 Cup of Celery, Thinly Sliced

-1 Cup of Walnuts, Chopped Finely

-2 Apples, Medium In Size, Ripe, Closed and Sliced Thinly

Directions:

1. Using a small sized mixing bowl combine your lemon juice, dash of salt, dash of pepper, coconut milk and tahini until well combined.

2. Then divide your lettuce evenly between four serving plates. In a separate mixing bowl combine your celery, nuts and apples together until evenly mixes. Toss with your freshly made dressing until evenly coated and top your salad with your walnut mixture.

Healthy Spinach Salad With Some Fresh Eggs and Bacon

This is another hearty salad that will soon become a fan favorite in your household. With the Bacon and the eggs this dish is one unique salad with a few favorite extra thrown in for a delicious dish.

Makes: 2 Plates

Ingredients:

-3 Slices of Cooked Bacon, Thick Cut

-2 Tbsp. of Olive Oil, Extra Virgin

-2 Tbsp. of Vinegar, Red Wine

-Dash of Dry Mustard Powder

-Dash of Salt For Taste

-1 Egg, Hardboiled, Peeled and Finely Chopped

-4 Cups of Baby Spinach, Fresh

-1/4 Cup of Red Onion, Sliced Thinly

Directions:

1. Using a medium sized skillet add in your olive oil, mustard powder, dash of salt, vinegar and cooked bacon. Whisk mixture over medium heat until smooth in consistency. Remove from heat.

2. Using a large sized mixing bowl combine your spinach and red onion together until thoroughly mixed.

3. Then drizzle your fresh dressing on top and toss salad until evenly coated. Pour onto 2 serving plates and top with your eggs. Serve and enjoy.

Conclusion

Hopefully you have found some of the best Paleo friendly recipes that you will ever lay your eyes on. There are plenty of Paleo style breakfast, lunch, dinner and dessert recipes here that you can make to impress your friends or family.

I know that being on a Paleo diet can seem like a torture spell and a punishment for you, but that could not be any further from the truth. As long as you try your best to spice up your dish and remember to use as many fruits and veggies as possible, all of the dishes that you can make with the help of this cookbook will be the healthiest and most nutritious meals that you can possibly make.

About Us:

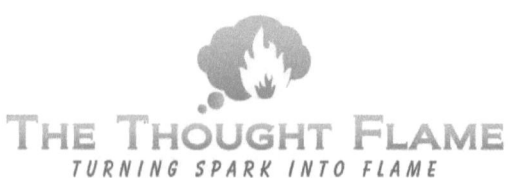

The Thought Flame is committed to add value to its customers through various books, online courses and other resources. You can learn more about us and our books at www.thethoughtflame.com.

Don't forget to check out our amazing **online video courses** at www.thethoughtflame.com/courses/ to take your knowledge to another level.

To check out our **extraordinary collection of diet/cookbooks**, visit http://www.thethoughtflame.com/category/non-fictional/cookbooks/ .

As a part of our valued relationship with our customers, we keep providing you free promotional books, courses and other stuff on subscribing with us on our site. We have a strict anti-spam policy and assure you no spam mails will be sent to your mailbox.

To subscribe with us, visit
www.thethoughtflame.com.

Like our work and would like to say thanks?

Buy us a cup of coffee at
www.thethoughtflame.com/coffee/

Author:

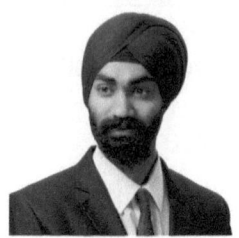

Amarpreet Singh is an avid learner and his passion for education has made him travel, work and study all across the world. He holds three masters degrees, including MBA, from top universities in Asia.

He is author of dozens of books, many of which are Amazon's bestseller, varying in various topics and categories. He also teaches many online courses having thousands of students across the world.

He has a keen interest in international affairs, economics, global poverty and politics, financial markets and entrepreneurship, and strives to be part of a community that shares the same passion.

He has worked as consultant with organizations like Airbus and The World Bank.

He loves travelling and learning about new cultures, and has been fortunate to live/work/travel/study in countries like India, China, Korea, US, South Africa, Japan, Philippines, Singapore, Canada etc., and learn about the culture and lifestyle in each of them.

To check out more of his work, visit www.thethoughtflame.com